Copyright 2022 - All rights reserved.

You may not reproduce, duplicate or send the contents of this book without direct written permission from the author. You cannot apply hereby despite any circumstance blame the publisher or hold him or her to legal responsibility for any reparation, compensations, or monetary forfeiture owing to the information included herein, either in a direct or an indirect way.

Legal Notice: This book has copyright protection. You can use the book for personal purposes. You should not sell, use, alter, distribute, quote, take excerpts, or paraphrase in part or whole the material contained in this book without obtaining the permission of the author first.

Disclaimer Notice: You must take note that the information in this document is for casual reading and entertainment purposes only. We have made every attempt to provide accurate, up-to-date, and reliable information. We do not express or imply guarantees of any kind. The persons who read admit that the writer is not occupied in giving legal, financial, medical, or other advice. We put this book content by sourcing various places.

Please consult a licensed professional before you try any techniques shown in this book. By going through this document, the book lover comes to an an agreement that under no situation is the author accountable for any forfeiture, direct or indirect, which they may incur because of the use of material contained in this document, including, but not limited to, — errors, omissions, or inaccuracies.

Personal Data

Name _____
Phone _____
Adress _____

In case of emergency
Please contavt

Name _____
Phone _____
Adress _____

Essential Contacts

Doctor _____
Pharmacy _____
Eye Clinic _____
Dentist _____

Name _____	**Name** _____
Cell: _____	Cell: _____
Work: _____	Work: _____
Home: _____	Home: _____
Email: _____	Email: _____
Others: _____	Others: _____

Notes

_____
_____
_____
_____
_____

> ....

Month: ....
Year: ....

Date	Time	SYS / DIA	Blood Pressure /	Heart Rate /	Respiratory Rate /	Oxygen Level /	Blood Sugar (Pre/Post Meal or Fasting)	°C / °F	Temperature /	Weight	Notes
	○am. ○pm.						○Pre○Post○FBS				
Notes:											
	○am. ○pm.						○Pre○Post○FBS				
Notes:											
	○am. ○pm.						○Pre○Post○FBS				
Notes:											
	○am. ○pm.						○Pre○Post○FBS				
Notes:											
	○am. ○pm.						○Pre○Post○FBS				
Notes:											
	○am. ○pm.						○Pre○Post○FBS				
Notes:											
	○am. ○pm.						○Pre○Post○FBS				
Notes:											
	○am. ○pm.						○Pre○Post○FBS				
Notes:											
	○am. ○pm.						○Pre○Post○FBS				
Notes:											
	○am. ○pm.						○Pre○Post○FBS				
Notes:											
	○am. ○pm.						○Pre○Post○FBS				
Notes:											
	○am. ○pm.						○Pre○Post○FBS				
Notes:											
	○am. ○pm.						○Pre○Post○FBS				
Notes:											
	○am. ○pm.						○Pre○Post○FBS				
Notes:											
	○am. ○pm.						○Pre○Post○FBS				

> ....

Month:........................
Year:..........................

Date	Time	SYS / DIA	Blood Pressure	Heart Rate	Respiratory Rate	Oxygen Level	Blood Sugar (Pre/Post Meal or Fasting)	Temperature °C/°F	Weight	Notes
	○am. ○pm.	/					○Pre ○Post ○FBS	/		
Notes:										
	○am. ○pm.	/					○Pre ○Post ○FBS	/		
Notes:										
	○am. ○pm.	/					○Pre ○Post ○FBS	/		
Notes:										
	○am. ○pm.	/					○Pre ○Post ○FBS	/		
Notes:										
	○am. ○pm.	/					○Pre ○Post ○FBS	/		
Notes:										
	○am. ○pm.	/					○Pre ○Post ○FBS	/		
Notes:										
	○am. ○pm.	/					○Pre ○Post ○FBS	/		
Notes:										
	○am. ○pm.	/					○Pre ○Post ○FBS	/		
Notes:										
	○am. ○pm.	/					○Pre ○Post ○FBS	/		
Notes:										
	○am. ○pm.	/					○Pre ○Post ○FBS	/		
Notes:										
	○am. ○pm.	/					○Pre ○Post ○FBS	/		
Notes:										
	○am. ○pm.	/					○Pre ○Post ○FBS	/		
Notes:										
	○am. ○pm.	/					○Pre ○Post ○FBS	/		
Notes:										
	○am. ○pm.	/					○Pre ○Post ○FBS	/		
Notes:										
	○am. ○pm.	/					○Pre ○Post ○FBS	/		
Notes:										
	○am. ○pm.	/					○Pre ○Post ○FBS	/		

> ....

Month: ....
Year: ....

Date	Time	SYS / DIA	Blood Pressure	Heart Rate	Respiratory Rate	Oxygen Level	Blood Sugar (Pre/Post Meal or Fasting)	Temperature °C/°F	Weight	Notes
	○am. ○pm.	/					○Pre ○Post ○FBS			
Notes:										
	○am. ○pm.	/					○Pre ○Post ○FBS			
Notes:										
	○am. ○pm.	/					○Pre ○Post ○FBS			
Notes:										
	○am. ○pm.	/					○Pre ○Post ○FBS			
Notes:										
	○am. ○pm.	/					○Pre ○Post ○FBS			
Notes:										
	○am. ○pm.	/					○Pre ○Post ○FBS			
Notes:										
	○am. ○pm.	/					○Pre ○Post ○FBS			
Notes:										
	○am. ○pm.	/					○Pre ○Post ○FBS			
Notes:										
	○am. ○pm.	/					○Pre ○Post ○FBS			
Notes:										
	○am. ○pm.	/					○Pre ○Post ○FBS			
Notes:										
	○am. ○pm.	/					○Pre ○Post ○FBS			
Notes:										
	○am. ○pm.	/					○Pre ○Post ○FBS			
Notes:										
	○am. ○pm.	/					○Pre ○Post ○FBS			
Notes:										
	○am. ○pm.	/					○Pre ○Post ○FBS			
Notes:										
	○am. ○pm.	/					○Pre ○Post ○FBS			
Notes:										
	○am. ○pm.	/					○Pre ○Post ○FBS			

> ....

Month: ....
Year: ....

Date	Time	SYS / DIA	Blood Pressure	Heart Rate	Respiratory Rate	Oxygen Level	Blood Sugar (Pre/Post Meal or Fasting)	Temperature °C/°F	Weight	Notes
	○am. ○pm.	/					○Pre ○Post ○FBS	/		
Notes:										
	○am. ○pm.	/					○Pre ○Post ○FBS	/		
Notes:										
	○am. ○pm.	/					○Pre ○Post ○FBS	/		
Notes:										
	○am. ○pm.	/					○Pre ○Post ○FBS	/		
Notes:										
	○am. ○pm.	/					○Pre ○Post ○FBS	/		
Notes:										
	○am. ○pm.	/					○Pre ○Post ○FBS	/		
Notes:										
	○am. ○pm.	/					○Pre ○Post ○FBS	/		
Notes:										
	○am. ○pm.	/					○Pre ○Post ○FBS	/		
Notes:										
	○am. ○pm.	/					○Pre ○Post ○FBS	/		
Notes:										
	○am. ○pm.	/					○Pre ○Post ○FBS	/		
Notes:										
	○am. ○pm.	/					○Pre ○Post ○FBS	/		
Notes:										
	○am. ○pm.	/					○Pre ○Post ○FBS	/		
Notes:										
	○am. ○pm.	/					○Pre ○Post ○FBS	/		
Notes:										
	○am. ○pm.	/					○Pre ○Post ○FBS	/		
Notes:										
	○am. ○pm.	/					○Pre ○Post ○FBS	/		
Notes:										
	○am. ○pm.	/					○Pre ○Post ○FBS	/		

> ....

Month:......................
Year:......................

Date	Time	SYS / DIA	Blood Pressure	Heart Rate	Respiratory Rate	Oxygen Level	Blood Sugar (Pre/Post Meal or Fasting)	Temperature °C/°F	Weight	Notes
	○am. ○pm.						○Pre ○Post ○FBS			
Notes:										
	○am. ○pm.						○Pre ○Post ○FBS			
Notes:										
	○am. ○pm.						○Pre ○Post ○FBS			
Notes:										
	○am. ○pm.						○Pre ○Post ○FBS			
Notes:										
	○am. ○pm.						○Pre ○Post ○FBS			
Notes:										
	○am. ○pm.						○Pre ○Post ○FBS			
Notes:										
	○am. ○pm.						○Pre ○Post ○FBS			
Notes:										
	○am. ○pm.						○Pre ○Post ○FBS			
Notes:										
	○am. ○pm.						○Pre ○Post ○FBS			
Notes:										
	○am. ○pm.						○Pre ○Post ○FBS			
Notes:										
	○am. ○pm.						○Pre ○Post ○FBS			
Notes:										
	○am. ○pm.						○Pre ○Post ○FBS			
Notes:										
	○am. ○pm.						○Pre ○Post ○FBS			
Notes:										
	○am. ○pm.						○Pre ○Post ○FBS			
Notes:										
	○am. ○pm.						○Pre ○Post ○FBS			
Notes:										
	○am. ○pm.						○Pre ○Post ○FBS			

> ....

Month: ....
Year: ....

Date	Time	Blood Pressure SYS / DIA	Heart Rate	Respiratory Rate	Oxygen Level	Blood Sugar (Pre/Post Meal or Fasting)	Temperature °C / °F	Weight	Notes
	○am. ○pm.	/				○Pre ○Post ○FBS	/		
Notes:									
	○am. ○pm.	/				○Pre ○Post ○FBS	/		
Notes:									
	○am. ○pm.	/				○Pre ○Post ○FBS	/		
Notes:									
	○am. ○pm.	/				○Pre ○Post ○FBS	/		
Notes:									
	○am. ○pm.	/				○Pre ○Post ○FBS	/		
Notes:									
	○am. ○pm.	/				○Pre ○Post ○FBS	/		
Notes:									
	○am. ○pm.	/				○Pre ○Post ○FBS	/		
Notes:									
	○am. ○pm.	/				○Pre ○Post ○FBS	/		
Notes:									
	○am. ○pm.	/				○Pre ○Post ○FBS	/		
Notes:									
	○am. ○pm.	/				○Pre ○Post ○FBS	/		
Notes:									
	○am. ○pm.	/				○Pre ○Post ○FBS	/		
Notes:									
	○am. ○pm.	/				○Pre ○Post ○FBS	/		
Notes:									
	○am. ○pm.	/				○Pre ○Post ○FBS	/		
Notes:									
	○am. ○pm.	/				○Pre ○Post ○FBS	/		
Notes:									
	○am. ○pm.	/				○Pre ○Post ○FBS	/		
Notes:									
	○am. ○pm.	/				○Pre ○Post ○FBS	/		

Medication Information

Date	Medication	Notes

Medication Information

Date	Medication	Notes

Medication Information

Date	Medication	Notes

Notes

Notes

Notes

Notes

Notes

> ....

Month:........................
Year:........................

Date	Time	SYS / DIA	Blood Pressure /	Heart Rate /	Respiratory Rate /	Oxygen Level /	Blood Sugar (Pre/Post Meal or Fasting)	Temperature °C / °F	Weight /	Notes
	○am. ○pm.						○Pre○Post○FBS			
Notes:										
	○am. ○pm.						○Pre○Post○FBS			
Notes:										
	○am. ○pm.						○Pre○Post○FBS			
Notes:										
	○am. ○pm.						○Pre○Post○FBS			
Notes:										
	○am. ○pm.						○Pre○Post○FBS			
Notes:										
	○am. ○pm.						○Pre○Post○FBS			
Notes:										
	○am. ○pm.						○Pre○Post○FBS			
Notes:										
	○am. ○pm.						○Pre○Post○FBS			
Notes:										
	○am. ○pm.						○Pre○Post○FBS			
Notes:										
	○am. ○pm.						○Pre○Post○FBS			
Notes:										
	○am. ○pm.						○Pre○Post○FBS			
Notes:										
	○am. ○pm.						○Pre○Post○FBS			
Notes:										
	○am. ○pm.						○Pre○Post○FBS			
Notes:										
	○am. ○pm.						○Pre○Post○FBS			
Notes:										
	○am. ○pm.						○Pre○Post○FBS			
Notes:										
	○am. ○pm.						○Pre○Post○FBS			

> ....

Month: ....
Year: ....

Date	Time	SYS / DIA	Blood Pressure	Heart Rate	Respiratory Rate	Oxygen Level	Blood Sugar (Pre/Post Meal or Fasting)	Temperature °C / °F	Weight	Notes
	○am. ○pm.						○Pre ○Post ○FBS			
Notes:										
	○am. ○pm.						○Pre ○Post ○FBS			
Notes:										
	○am. ○pm.						○Pre ○Post ○FBS			
Notes:										
	○am. ○pm.						○Pre ○Post ○FBS			
Notes:										
	○am. ○pm.						○Pre ○Post ○FBS			
Notes:										
	○am. ○pm.						○Pre ○Post ○FBS			
Notes:										
	○am. ○pm.						○Pre ○Post ○FBS			
Notes:										
	○am. ○pm.						○Pre ○Post ○FBS			
Notes:										
	○am. ○pm.						○Pre ○Post ○FBS			
Notes:										
	○am. ○pm.						○Pre ○Post ○FBS			
Notes:										
	○am. ○pm.						○Pre ○Post ○FBS			
Notes:										
	○am. ○pm.						○Pre ○Post ○FBS			
Notes:										
	○am. ○pm.						○Pre ○Post ○FBS			
Notes:										
	○am. ○pm.						○Pre ○Post ○FBS			
Notes:										
	○am. ○pm.						○Pre ○Post ○FBS			
Notes:										
	○am. ○pm.						○Pre ○Post ○FBS			

> ....

Month:........................
Year:........................

Date	Time	Blood Pressure SYS / DIA	Heart Rate	Respiratory Rate	Oxygen Level	Blood Sugar (Pre/Post Meal or Fasting)	Temperature °C/°F	Weight	Notes
	○am. ○pm.	/				○Pre ○Post ○FBS	/		
Notes:									
	○am. ○pm.	/				○Pre ○Post ○FBS	/		
Notes:									
	○am. ○pm.	/				○Pre ○Post ○FBS	/		
Notes:									
	○am. ○pm.	/				○Pre ○Post ○FBS	/		
Notes:									
	○am. ○pm.	/				○Pre ○Post ○FBS	/		
Notes:									
	○am. ○pm.	/				○Pre ○Post ○FBS	/		
Notes:									
	○am. ○pm.	/				○Pre ○Post ○FBS	/		
Notes:									
	○am. ○pm.	/				○Pre ○Post ○FBS	/		
Notes:									
	○am. ○pm.	/				○Pre ○Post ○FBS	/		
Notes:									
	○am. ○pm.	/				○Pre ○Post ○FBS	/		
Notes:									
	○am. ○pm.	/				○Pre ○Post ○FBS	/		
Notes:									
	○am. ○pm.	/				○Pre ○Post ○FBS	/		
Notes:									
	○am. ○pm.	/				○Pre ○Post ○FBS	/		
Notes:									
	○am. ○pm.	/				○Pre ○Post ○FBS	/		
Notes:									
	○am. ○pm.	/				○Pre ○Post ○FBS	/		

> ....

Month:........................
Year:........................

Date	Time	SYS / DIA	Blood Pressure /	Heart Rate /	Respiratory Rate /	Oxygen Level /	Blood Sugar (Pre/Post Meal or Fasting)	°C / °F	Temperature / Weight	Notes
	○am. ○pm.						○Pre○Post○FBS			
Notes:										
	○am. ○pm.						○Pre○Post○FBS			
Notes:										
	○am. ○pm.						○Pre○Post○FBS			
Notes:										
	○am. ○pm.						○Pre○Post○FBS			
Notes:										
	○am. ○pm.						○Pre○Post○FBS			
Notes:										
	○am. ○pm.						○Pre○Post○FBS			
Notes:										
	○am. ○pm.						○Pre○Post○FBS			
Notes:										
	○am. ○pm.						○Pre○Post○FBS			
Notes:										
	○am. ○pm.						○Pre○Post○FBS			
Notes:										
	○am. ○pm.						○Pre○Post○FBS			
Notes:										
	○am. ○pm.						○Pre○Post○FBS			
Notes:										
	○am. ○pm.						○Pre○Post○FBS			
Notes:										
	○am. ○pm.						○Pre○Post○FBS			
Notes:										
	○am. ○pm.						○Pre○Post○FBS			
Notes:										
	○am. ○pm.						○Pre○Post○FBS			
Notes:										
	○am. ○pm.						○Pre○Post○FBS			

> ....

Month:........................
Year:........................

Date	Time	SYS / DIA	Blood Pressure /	Heart Rate /	Respiratory Rate /	Oxygen Level /	Blood Sugar (Pre/Post Meal or Fasting)	Temperature °C/°F /	Weight	Notes
	○am. ○pm.						○Pre○Post○FBS			
Notes:										
	○am. ○pm.						○Pre○Post○FBS			
Notes:										
	○am. ○pm.						○Pre○Post○FBS			
Notes:										
	○am. ○pm.						○Pre○Post○FBS			
Notes:										
	○am. ○pm.						○Pre○Post○FBS			
Notes:										
	○am. ○pm.						○Pre○Post○FBS			
Notes:										
	○am. ○pm.						○Pre○Post○FBS			
Notes:										
	○am. ○pm.						○Pre○Post○FBS			
Notes:										
	○am. ○pm.						○Pre○Post○FBS			
Notes:										
	○am. ○pm.						○Pre○Post○FBS			
Notes:										
	○am. ○pm.						○Pre○Post○FBS			
Notes:										
	○am. ○pm.						○Pre○Post○FBS			
Notes:										
	○am. ○pm.						○Pre○Post○FBS			
Notes:										
	○am. ○pm.						○Pre○Post○FBS			
Notes:										
	○am. ○pm.						○Pre○Post○FBS			
Notes:										
	○am. ○pm.						○Pre○Post○FBS			

>

Month:..........................
Year:...........................

Date	Time	SYS / DIA	Blood Pressure /	Heart Rate /	Respiratory Rate /	Oxygen Level /	Blood Sugar (Pre/Post Meal or Fasting)	Temperature °C/°F /	Weight	Notes
	○am. ○pm.						○Pre ○Post ○FBS			
Notes:										
	○am. ○pm.						○Pre ○Post ○FBS			
Notes:										
	○am. ○pm.						○Pre ○Post ○FBS			
Notes:										
	○am. ○pm.						○Pre ○Post ○FBS			
Notes:										
	○am. ○pm.						○Pre ○Post ○FBS			
Notes:										
	○am. ○pm.						○Pre ○Post ○FBS			
Notes:										
	○am. ○pm.						○Pre ○Post ○FBS			
Notes:										
	○am. ○pm.						○Pre ○Post ○FBS			
Notes:										
	○am. ○pm.						○Pre ○Post ○FBS			
Notes:										
	○am. ○pm.						○Pre ○Post ○FBS			
Notes:										
	○am. ○pm.						○Pre ○Post ○FBS			
Notes:										
	○am. ○pm.						○Pre ○Post ○FBS			
Notes:										
	○am. ○pm.						○Pre ○Post ○FBS			
Notes:										
	○am. ○pm.						○Pre ○Post ○FBS			
Notes:										
	○am. ○pm.						○Pre ○Post ○FBS			
Notes:										
	○am. ○pm.						○Pre ○Post ○FBS			

Medication Information

Date	Medication	Notes

Medication Information

Date	Medication	Notes

Medication Information

Date	Medication	Notes

Notes

Notes

Notes

Notes

Notes

> ....

Month:........................
Year:.........................

Date	Time	SYS / DIA	Blood Pressure /	Heart Rate /	Respiratory Rate /	Oxygen Level /	Blood Sugar (Pre/Post Meal or Fasting)	Temperature °C/°F /	Weight	Notes
	○am. ○pm.						○Pre○Post○FBS			
Notes:										
	○am. ○pm.						○Pre○Post○FBS			
Notes:										
	○am. ○pm.						○Pre○Post○FBS			
Notes:										
	○am. ○pm.						○Pre○Post○FBS			
Notes:										
	○am. ○pm.						○Pre○Post○FBS			
Notes:										
	○am. ○pm.						○Pre○Post○FBS			
Notes:										
	○am. ○pm.						○Pre○Post○FBS			
Notes:										
	○am. ○pm.						○Pre○Post○FBS			
Notes:										
	○am. ○pm.						○Pre○Post○FBS			
Notes:										
	○am. ○pm.						○Pre○Post○FBS			
Notes:										
	○am. ○pm.						○Pre○Post○FBS			
Notes:										
	○am. ○pm.						○Pre○Post○FBS			
Notes:										
	○am. ○pm.						○Pre○Post○FBS			
Notes:										
	○am. ○pm.						○Pre○Post○FBS			
Notes:										
	○am. ○pm.						○Pre○Post○FBS			
Notes:										
	○am. ○pm.						○Pre○Post○FBS			

>..

Month:........................
Year:........................

Date	Time	SYS / DIA	Blood Pressure /	Heart Rate /	Respiratory Rate /	Oxygen Level /	Blood Sugar (Pre/Post Meal or Fasting)	°C / °F	Temperature / Weight	Notes
	○am. ○pm.						○Pre○Post○FBS			
Notes:										
	○am. ○pm.						○Pre○Post○FBS			
Notes:										
	○am. ○pm.						○Pre○Post○FBS			
Notes:										
	○am. ○pm.						○Pre○Post○FBS			
Notes:										
	○am. ○pm.						○Pre○Post○FBS			
Notes:										
	○am. ○pm.						○Pre○Post○FBS			
Notes:										
	○am. ○pm.						○Pre○Post○FBS			
Notes:										
	○am. ○pm.						○Pre○Post○FBS			
Notes:										
	○am. ○pm.						○Pre○Post○FBS			
Notes:										
	○am. ○pm.						○Pre○Post○FBS			
Notes:										
	○am. ○pm.						○Pre○Post○FBS			
Notes:										
	○am. ○pm.						○Pre○Post○FBS			
Notes:										
	○am. ○pm.						○Pre○Post○FBS			
Notes:										
	○am. ○pm.						○Pre○Post○FBS			
Notes:										
	○am. ○pm.						○Pre○Post○FBS			
Notes:										
	○am. ○pm.						○Pre○Post○FBS			

> ....

Month:........................
Year:........................

Date	Time	SYS / DIA	Blood Pressure	Heart Rate	Respiratory Rate	Oxygen Level	Blood Sugar (Pre/Post Meal or Fasting)	Temperature °C/°F	Weight	Notes
	○am. ○pm.						○Pre○Post○FBS			
Notes:										
	○am. ○pm.						○Pre○Post○FBS			
Notes:										
	○am. ○pm.						○Pre○Post○FBS			
Notes:										
	○am. ○pm.						○Pre○Post○FBS			
Notes:										
	○am. ○pm.						○Pre○Post○FBS			
Notes:										
	○am. ○pm.						○Pre○Post○FBS			
Notes:										
	○am. ○pm.						○Pre○Post○FBS			
Notes:										
	○am. ○pm.						○Pre○Post○FBS			
Notes:										
	○am. ○pm.						○Pre○Post○FBS			
Notes:										
	○am. ○pm.						○Pre○Post○FBS			
Notes:										
	○am. ○pm.						○Pre○Post○FBS			
Notes:										
	○am. ○pm.						○Pre○Post○FBS			
Notes:										
	○am. ○pm.						○Pre○Post○FBS			
Notes:										
	○am. ○pm.						○Pre○Post○FBS			
Notes:										
	○am. ○pm.						○Pre○Post○FBS			
Notes:										
	○am. ○pm.						○Pre○Post○FBS			

>..

Month:........................
Year:........................

Date	Time	Blood Pressure SYS / DIA	Heart Rate /	Respiratory Rate /	Oxygen Level /	Blood Sugar (Pre/Post Meal or Fasting)	Temperature °C / °F	Weight /	Notes
	○am. ○pm.	|				○Pre○Post○FBS			
Notes:									
	○am. ○pm.	|				○Pre○Post○FBS			
Notes:									
	○am. ○pm.	|				○Pre○Post○FBS			
Notes:									
	○am. ○pm.	|				○Pre○Post○FBS			
Notes:									
	○am. ○pm.	|				○Pre○Post○FBS			
Notes:									
	○am. ○pm.	|				○Pre○Post○FBS			
Notes:									
	○am. ○pm.	|				○Pre○Post○FBS			
Notes:									
	○am. ○pm.	|				○Pre○Post○FBS			
Notes:									
	○am. ○pm.	|				○Pre○Post○FBS			
Notes:									
	○am. ○pm.	|				○Pre○Post○FBS			
Notes:									
	○am. ○pm.	|				○Pre○Post○FBS			
Notes:									
	○am. ○pm.	|				○Pre○Post○FBS			
Notes:									
	○am. ○pm.	|				○Pre○Post○FBS			
Notes:									
	○am. ○pm.	|				○Pre○Post○FBS			
Notes:									
	○am. ○pm.	|				○Pre○Post○FBS			

> ....

Month:......................
Year:........................

Date	Time	SYS / DIA	Blood Pressure /	Heart Rate /	Respiratory Rate /	Oxygen Level /	Blood Sugar (Pre/Post Meal or Fasting)	Temperature °C / °F	Weight /	Notes
	○am. ○pm.						○Pre○Post○FBS			
Notes:										
	○am. ○pm.						○Pre○Post○FBS			
Notes:										
	○am. ○pm.						○Pre○Post○FBS			
Notes:										
	○am. ○pm.						○Pre○Post○FBS			
Notes:										
	○am. ○pm.						○Pre○Post○FBS			
Notes:										
	○am. ○pm.						○Pre○Post○FBS			
Notes:										
	○am. ○pm.						○Pre○Post○FBS			
Notes:										
	○am. ○pm.						○Pre○Post○FBS			
Notes:										
	○am. ○pm.						○Pre○Post○FBS			
Notes:										
	○am. ○pm.						○Pre○Post○FBS			
Notes:										
	○am. ○pm.						○Pre○Post○FBS			
Notes:										
	○am. ○pm.						○Pre○Post○FBS			
Notes:										
	○am. ○pm.						○Pre○Post○FBS			
Notes:										
	○am. ○pm.						○Pre○Post○FBS			
Notes:										
	○am. ○pm.						○Pre○Post○FBS			
Notes:										
	○am. ○pm.						○Pre○Post○FBS			

> ....

Month:........................
Year:........................

Date	Time	SYS / DIA	Blood Pressure /	Heart Rate /	Respiratory Rate /	Oxygen Level /	Blood Sugar (Pre/Post Meal or Fasting)	°C / °F	Temperature / Weight	Notes
	○am. ○pm.						○Pre○Post○FBS			
Notes:										
	○am. ○pm.						○Pre○Post○FBS			
Notes:										
	○am. ○pm.						○Pre○Post○FBS			
Notes:										
	○am. ○pm.						○Pre○Post○FBS			
Notes:										
	○am. ○pm.						○Pre○Post○FBS			
Notes:										
	○am. ○pm.						○Pre○Post○FBS			
Notes:										
	○am. ○pm.						○Pre○Post○FBS			
Notes:										
	○am. ○pm.						○Pre○Post○FBS			
Notes:										
	○am. ○pm.						○Pre○Post○FBS			
Notes:										
	○am. ○pm.						○Pre○Post○FBS			
Notes:										
	○am. ○pm.						○Pre○Post○FBS			
Notes:										
	○am. ○pm.						○Pre○Post○FBS			
Notes:										
	○am. ○pm.						○Pre○Post○FBS			
Notes:										
	○am. ○pm.						○Pre○Post○FBS			
Notes:										
	○am. ○pm.						○Pre○Post○FBS			
Notes:										
	○am. ○pm.						○Pre○Post○FBS			

Medication Information

Date	Medication	Notes

Medication Information

Date	Medication	Notes

Medication Information

Date	Medication	Notes

Notes

Notes

Notes

Notes

Notes

>
....

Month:........................
Year:........................

Date	Time	Blood Pressure SYS / DIA	Heart Rate	Respiratory Rate	Oxygen Level	Blood Sugar (Pre/Post Meal or Fasting)	Temperature °C / °F	Weight	Notes
	○am. ○pm.	/				○Pre ○Post ○FBS	/		
Notes:									
	○am. ○pm.	/				○Pre ○Post ○FBS	/		
Notes:									
	○am. ○pm.	/				○Pre ○Post ○FBS	/		
Notes:									
	○am. ○pm.	/				○Pre ○Post ○FBS	/		
Notes:									
	○am. ○pm.	/				○Pre ○Post ○FBS	/		
Notes:									
	○am. ○pm.	/				○Pre ○Post ○FBS	/		
Notes:									
	○am. ○pm.	/				○Pre ○Post ○FBS	/		
Notes:									
	○am. ○pm.	/				○Pre ○Post ○FBS	/		
Notes:									
	○am. ○pm.	/				○Pre ○Post ○FBS	/		
Notes:									
	○am. ○pm.	/				○Pre ○Post ○FBS	/		
Notes:									
	○am. ○pm.	/				○Pre ○Post ○FBS	/		
Notes:									
	○am. ○pm.	/				○Pre ○Post ○FBS	/		
Notes:									
	○am. ○pm.	/				○Pre ○Post ○FBS	/		
Notes:									
	○am. ○pm.	/				○Pre ○Post ○FBS	/		
Notes:									
	○am. ○pm.	/				○Pre ○Post ○FBS	/		
Notes:									
	○am. ○pm.	/				○Pre ○Post ○FBS	/		

> ....

Month:..........................
Year:..........................

Date	Time	SYS / DIA	Blood Pressure	Heart Rate	Respiratory Rate	Oxygen Level	Blood Sugar (Pre/Post Meal or Fasting)	Temperature °C / °F	Weight	Notes
	○am. ○pm.						○Pre ○Post ○FBS			
Notes:										
	○am. ○pm.						○Pre ○Post ○FBS			
Notes:										
	○am. ○pm.						○Pre ○Post ○FBS			
Notes:										
	○am. ○pm.						○Pre ○Post ○FBS			
Notes:										
	○am. ○pm.						○Pre ○Post ○FBS			
Notes:										
	○am. ○pm.						○Pre ○Post ○FBS			
Notes:										
	○am. ○pm.						○Pre ○Post ○FBS			
Notes:										
	○am. ○pm.						○Pre ○Post ○FBS			
Notes:										
	○am. ○pm.						○Pre ○Post ○FBS			
Notes:										
	○am. ○pm.						○Pre ○Post ○FBS			
Notes:										
	○am. ○pm.						○Pre ○Post ○FBS			
Notes:										
	○am. ○pm.						○Pre ○Post ○FBS			
Notes:										
	○am. ○pm.						○Pre ○Post ○FBS			
Notes:										
	○am. ○pm.						○Pre ○Post ○FBS			
Notes:										
	○am. ○pm.						○Pre ○Post ○FBS			
Notes:										
	○am. ○pm.						○Pre ○Post ○FBS			

> ....

Month:........................
Year:........................

Date	Time	Blood Pressure SYS / DIA	Heart Rate	Respiratory Rate	Oxygen Level	Blood Sugar (Pre/Post Meal or Fasting)	Temperature °C / °F	Weight	Notes
	○am. ○pm.	/				○Pre ○Post ○FBS	/		
Notes:									
	○am. ○pm.	/				○Pre ○Post ○FBS	/		
Notes:									
	○am. ○pm.	/				○Pre ○Post ○FBS	/		
Notes:									
	○am. ○pm.	/				○Pre ○Post ○FBS	/		
Notes:									
	○am. ○pm.	/				○Pre ○Post ○FBS	/		
Notes:									
	○am. ○pm.	/				○Pre ○Post ○FBS	/		
Notes:									
	○am. ○pm.	/				○Pre ○Post ○FBS	/		
Notes:									
	○am. ○pm.	/				○Pre ○Post ○FBS	/		
Notes:									
	○am. ○pm.	/				○Pre ○Post ○FBS	/		
Notes:									
	○am. ○pm.	/				○Pre ○Post ○FBS	/		
Notes:									
	○am. ○pm.	/				○Pre ○Post ○FBS	/		
Notes:									
	○am. ○pm.	/				○Pre ○Post ○FBS	/		
Notes:									
	○am. ○pm.	/				○Pre ○Post ○FBS	/		
Notes:									
	○am. ○pm.	/				○Pre ○Post ○FBS	/		
Notes:									
	○am. ○pm.	/				○Pre ○Post ○FBS	/		
Notes:									
	○am. ○pm.	/				○Pre ○Post ○FBS	/		

Medication Information

Date	Medication	Notes

Medication Information

Date	Medication	Notes

Medication Information

Date	Medication	Notes

Notes

Notes

Notes

Notes

Notes

Notes

> ....

Month: ....
Year: ....

Date	Time	SYS / DIA	Blood Pressure	Heart Rate	Respiratory Rate	Oxygen Level	Blood Sugar (Pre/Post Meal or Fasting)	Temperature °C/°F	Weight	Notes
	○am. ○pm.						○Pre ○Post ○FBS			
Notes:										
	○am. ○pm.						○Pre ○Post ○FBS			
Notes:										
	○am. ○pm.						○Pre ○Post ○FBS			
Notes:										
	○am. ○pm.						○Pre ○Post ○FBS			
Notes:										
	○am. ○pm.						○Pre ○Post ○FBS			
Notes:										
	○am. ○pm.						○Pre ○Post ○FBS			
Notes:										
	○am. ○pm.						○Pre ○Post ○FBS			
Notes:										
	○am. ○pm.						○Pre ○Post ○FBS			
Notes:										
	○am. ○pm.						○Pre ○Post ○FBS			
Notes:										
	○am. ○pm.						○Pre ○Post ○FBS			
Notes:										
	○am. ○pm.						○Pre ○Post ○FBS			
Notes:										
	○am. ○pm.						○Pre ○Post ○FBS			
Notes:										
	○am. ○pm.						○Pre ○Post ○FBS			
Notes:										
	○am. ○pm.						○Pre ○Post ○FBS			
Notes:										
	○am. ○pm.						○Pre ○Post ○FBS			
Notes:										
	○am. ○pm.						○Pre ○Post ○FBS			

> ....

Month: ....
Year: ....

Date	Time	SYS / DIA	Blood Pressure	Heart Rate	Respiratory Rate	Oxygen Level	Blood Sugar (Pre/Post Meal or Fasting)	Temperature °C / °F	Weight	Notes
	○am. ○pm.						○Pre ○Post ○FBS			
Notes:										
	○am. ○pm.						○Pre ○Post ○FBS			
Notes:										
	○am. ○pm.						○Pre ○Post ○FBS			
Notes:										
	○am. ○pm.						○Pre ○Post ○FBS			
Notes:										
	○am. ○pm.						○Pre ○Post ○FBS			
Notes:										
	○am. ○pm.						○Pre ○Post ○FBS			
Notes:										
	○am. ○pm.						○Pre ○Post ○FBS			
Notes:										
	○am. ○pm.						○Pre ○Post ○FBS			
Notes:										
	○am. ○pm.						○Pre ○Post ○FBS			
Notes:										
	○am. ○pm.						○Pre ○Post ○FBS			
Notes:										
	○am. ○pm.						○Pre ○Post ○FBS			
Notes:										
	○am. ○pm.						○Pre ○Post ○FBS			
Notes:										
	○am. ○pm.						○Pre ○Post ○FBS			
Notes:										
	○am. ○pm.						○Pre ○Post ○FBS			
Notes:										
	○am. ○pm.						○Pre ○Post ○FBS			

> ....

Month:........................
Year:..........................

Date	Time	SYS / DIA	Blood Pressure /	Heart Rate /	Respiratory Rate /	Oxygen Level /	Blood Sugar (Pre/Post Meal or Fasting)	Temperature °C/°F /	Weight	Notes
	○am. ○pm.						○Pre○Post○FBS			
Notes:										
	○am. ○pm.						○Pre○Post○FBS			
Notes:										
	○am. ○pm.						○Pre○Post○FBS			
Notes:										
	○am. ○pm.						○Pre○Post○FBS			
Notes:										
	○am. ○pm.						○Pre○Post○FBS			
Notes:										
	○am. ○pm.						○Pre○Post○FBS			
Notes:										
	○am. ○pm.						○Pre○Post○FBS			
Notes:										
	○am. ○pm.						○Pre○Post○FBS			
Notes:										
	○am. ○pm.						○Pre○Post○FBS			
Notes:										
	○am. ○pm.						○Pre○Post○FBS			
Notes:										
	○am. ○pm.						○Pre○Post○FBS			
Notes:										
	○am. ○pm.						○Pre○Post○FBS			
Notes:										
	○am. ○pm.						○Pre○Post○FBS			
Notes:										
	○am. ○pm.						○Pre○Post○FBS			
Notes:										
	○am. ○pm.						○Pre○Post○FBS			
Notes:										
	○am. ○pm.						○Pre○Post○FBS			

> ....

Month:........................
Year:........................

Date	Time	Blood Pressure SYS / DIA	Heart Rate	Respiratory Rate	Oxygen Level	Blood Sugar (Pre/Post Meal or Fasting)	Temperature °C / °F	Weight	Notes
	○am. ○pm.	/				○Pre○Post○FBS	/		
Notes:									
	○am. ○pm.	/				○Pre○Post○FBS	/		
Notes:									
	○am. ○pm.	/				○Pre○Post○FBS	/		
Notes:									
	○am. ○pm.	/				○Pre○Post○FBS	/		
Notes:									
	○am. ○pm.	/				○Pre○Post○FBS	/		
Notes:									
	○am. ○pm.	/				○Pre○Post○FBS	/		
Notes:									
	○am. ○pm.	/				○Pre○Post○FBS	/		
Notes:									
	○am. ○pm.	/				○Pre○Post○FBS	/		
Notes:									
	○am. ○pm.	/				○Pre○Post○FBS	/		
Notes:									
	○am. ○pm.	/				○Pre○Post○FBS	/		
Notes:									
	○am. ○pm.	/				○Pre○Post○FBS	/		
Notes:									
	○am. ○pm.	/				○Pre○Post○FBS	/		
Notes:									
	○am. ○pm.	/				○Pre○Post○FBS	/		
Notes:									
	○am. ○pm.	/				○Pre○Post○FBS	/		
Notes:									
	○am. ○pm.	/				○Pre○Post○FBS	/		
Notes:									
	○am. ○pm.	/				○Pre○Post○FBS	/		

> ....

Month: ....
Year: ....

Date	Time	Blood Pressure SYS / DIA	Heart Rate	Respiratory Rate	Oxygen Level	Blood Sugar (Pre/Post Meal or Fasting)	Temperature °C / °F	Weight	Notes
	○am. ○pm.	/				○Pre ○Post ○FBS	/		
Notes:									
	○am. ○pm.	/				○Pre ○Post ○FBS	/		
Notes:									
	○am. ○pm.	/				○Pre ○Post ○FBS	/		
Notes:									
	○am. ○pm.	/				○Pre ○Post ○FBS	/		
Notes:									
	○am. ○pm.	/				○Pre ○Post ○FBS	/		
Notes:									
	○am. ○pm.	/				○Pre ○Post ○FBS	/		
Notes:									
	○am. ○pm.	/				○Pre ○Post ○FBS	/		
Notes:									
	○am. ○pm.	/				○Pre ○Post ○FBS	/		
Notes:									
	○am. ○pm.	/				○Pre ○Post ○FBS	/		
Notes:									
	○am. ○pm.	/				○Pre ○Post ○FBS	/		
Notes:									
	○am. ○pm.	/				○Pre ○Post ○FBS	/		
Notes:									
	○am. ○pm.	/				○Pre ○Post ○FBS	/		
Notes:									
	○am. ○pm.	/				○Pre ○Post ○FBS	/		
Notes:									
	○am. ○pm.	/				○Pre ○Post ○FBS	/		
Notes:									
	○am. ○pm.	/				○Pre ○Post ○FBS	/		
Notes:									
	○am. ○pm.	/				○Pre ○Post ○FBS	/		

> ....

Month: ....
Year: ....

Date	Time	SYS / DIA	Blood Pressure /	Heart Rate /	Respiratory Rate /	Oxygen Level /	Blood Sugar (Pre/Post Meal or Fasting)	Temperature °C/°F	Weight /	Notes
	○am. ○pm.					○Pre ○Post ○FBS				
Notes:										
	○am. ○pm.					○Pre ○Post ○FBS				
Notes:										
	○am. ○pm.					○Pre ○Post ○FBS				
Notes:										
	○am. ○pm.					○Pre ○Post ○FBS				
Notes:										
	○am. ○pm.					○Pre ○Post ○FBS				
Notes:										
	○am. ○pm.					○Pre ○Post ○FBS				
Notes:										
	○am. ○pm.					○Pre ○Post ○FBS				
Notes:										
	○am. ○pm.					○Pre ○Post ○FBS				
Notes:										
	○am. ○pm.					○Pre ○Post ○FBS				
Notes:										
	○am. ○pm.					○Pre ○Post ○FBS				
Notes:										
	○am. ○pm.					○Pre ○Post ○FBS				
Notes:										
	○am. ○pm.					○Pre ○Post ○FBS				
Notes:										
	○am. ○pm.					○Pre ○Post ○FBS				
Notes:										
	○am. ○pm.					○Pre ○Post ○FBS				
Notes:										
	○am. ○pm.					○Pre ○Post ○FBS				
Notes:										
	○am. ○pm.					○Pre ○Post ○FBS				

> ....

Month: ....
Year: ....

Date	Time	SYS / DIA Blood Pressure	Heart Rate	Respiratory Rate	Oxygen Level	Blood Sugar (Pre/Post Meal or Fasting)	Temperature °C / °F	Weight	Notes
	○am. ○pm.	/				○Pre ○Post ○FBS	/		
Notes:									
	○am. ○pm.	/				○Pre ○Post ○FBS	/		
Notes:									
	○am. ○pm.	/				○Pre ○Post ○FBS	/		
Notes:									
	○am. ○pm.	/				○Pre ○Post ○FBS	/		
Notes:									
	○am. ○pm.	/				○Pre ○Post ○FBS	/		
Notes:									
	○am. ○pm.	/				○Pre ○Post ○FBS	/		
Notes:									
	○am. ○pm.	/				○Pre ○Post ○FBS	/		
Notes:									
	○am. ○pm.	/				○Pre ○Post ○FBS	/		
Notes:									
	○am. ○pm.	/				○Pre ○Post ○FBS	/		
Notes:									
	○am. ○pm.	/				○Pre ○Post ○FBS	/		
Notes:									
	○am. ○pm.	/				○Pre ○Post ○FBS	/		
Notes:									
	○am. ○pm.	/				○Pre ○Post ○FBS	/		
Notes:									
	○am. ○pm.	/				○Pre ○Post ○FBS	/		
Notes:									
	○am. ○pm.	/				○Pre ○Post ○FBS	/		
Notes:									
	○am. ○pm.	/				○Pre ○Post ○FBS	/		
Notes:									
	○am. ○pm.	/				○Pre ○Post ○FBS	/		

Medication Information

Date	Medication	Notes

Medication Information

Date	Medication	Notes

Medication Information

Date	Medication	Notes

Notes

Notes

Notes

Notes

Notes

\>
....

Month:........................
Year:..........................

Date	Time	SYS / DIA	Blood Pressure	Heart Rate	Respiratory Rate	Oxygen Level	Blood Sugar (Pre/Post Meal or Fasting)	Temperature °C/°F	Weight	Notes
	○am. ○pm.						○Pre ○Post ○FBS			
Notes:										
	○am. ○pm.						○Pre ○Post ○FBS			
Notes:										
	○am. ○pm.						○Pre ○Post ○FBS			
Notes:										
	○am. ○pm.						○Pre ○Post ○FBS			
Notes:										
	○am. ○pm.						○Pre ○Post ○FBS			
Notes:										
	○am. ○pm.						○Pre ○Post ○FBS			
Notes:										
	○am. ○pm.						○Pre ○Post ○FBS			
Notes:										
	○am. ○pm.						○Pre ○Post ○FBS			
Notes:										
	○am. ○pm.						○Pre ○Post ○FBS			
Notes:										
	○am. ○pm.						○Pre ○Post ○FBS			
Notes:										
	○am. ○pm.						○Pre ○Post ○FBS			
Notes:										
	○am. ○pm.						○Pre ○Post ○FBS			
Notes:										
	○am. ○pm.						○Pre ○Post ○FBS			
Notes:										
	○am. ○pm.						○Pre ○Post ○FBS			
Notes:										
	○am. ○pm.						○Pre ○Post ○FBS			

> ....

Month:........................
Year:........................

Date	Time	SYS / DIA (Blood Pressure)	Heart Rate	Respiratory Rate	Oxygen Level	Blood Sugar (Pre/Post Meal or Fasting)	Temperature °C/°F	Weight	Notes
	○am. ○pm.	/				○Pre ○Post ○FBS	/		
Notes:									
	○am. ○pm.	/				○Pre ○Post ○FBS	/		
Notes:									
	○am. ○pm.	/				○Pre ○Post ○FBS	/		
Notes:									
	○am. ○pm.	/				○Pre ○Post ○FBS	/		
Notes:									
	○am. ○pm.	/				○Pre ○Post ○FBS	/		
Notes:									
	○am. ○pm.	/				○Pre ○Post ○FBS	/		
Notes:									
	○am. ○pm.	/				○Pre ○Post ○FBS	/		
Notes:									
	○am. ○pm.	/				○Pre ○Post ○FBS	/		
Notes:									
	○am. ○pm.	/				○Pre ○Post ○FBS	/		
Notes:									
	○am. ○pm.	/				○Pre ○Post ○FBS	/		
Notes:									
	○am. ○pm.	/				○Pre ○Post ○FBS	/		
Notes:									
	○am. ○pm.	/				○Pre ○Post ○FBS	/		
Notes:									
	○am. ○pm.	/				○Pre ○Post ○FBS	/		
Notes:									
	○am. ○pm.	/				○Pre ○Post ○FBS	/		
Notes:									
	○am. ○pm.	/				○Pre ○Post ○FBS	/		
Notes:									
	○am. ○pm.	/				○Pre ○Post ○FBS	/		

> ....

Month:........................
Year:........................

Date	Time	SYS / DIA	Blood Pressure /	Heart Rate /	Respiratory Rate /	Oxygen Level /	Blood Sugar (Pre/Post Meal or Fasting)	Temperature °C/°F /	Weight	Notes
	○am. ○pm.						○Pre ○Post ○FBS			
Notes:										
	○am. ○pm.						○Pre ○Post ○FBS			
Notes:										
	○am. ○pm.						○Pre ○Post ○FBS			
Notes:										
	○am. ○pm.						○Pre ○Post ○FBS			
Notes:										
	○am. ○pm.						○Pre ○Post ○FBS			
Notes:										
	○am. ○pm.						○Pre ○Post ○FBS			
Notes:										
	○am. ○pm.						○Pre ○Post ○FBS			
Notes:										
	○am. ○pm.						○Pre ○Post ○FBS			
Notes:										
	○am. ○pm.						○Pre ○Post ○FBS			
Notes:										
	○am. ○pm.						○Pre ○Post ○FBS			
Notes:										
	○am. ○pm.						○Pre ○Post ○FBS			
Notes:										
	○am. ○pm.						○Pre ○Post ○FBS			
Notes:										
	○am. ○pm.						○Pre ○Post ○FBS			
Notes:										
	○am. ○pm.						○Pre ○Post ○FBS			
Notes:										
	○am. ○pm.						○Pre ○Post ○FBS			

> ....

Month:......................
Year:........................

Date	Time	SYS / DIA	Blood Pressure /	Heart Rate /	Respiratory Rate /	Oxygen Level /	Blood Sugar (Pre/Post Meal or Fasting)	Temperature °C/°F	Weight /	Notes
	○am. ○pm.						○Pre○Post○FBS			
Notes:										
	○am. ○pm.						○Pre○Post○FBS			
Notes:										
	○am. ○pm.						○Pre○Post○FBS			
Notes:										
	○am. ○pm.						○Pre○Post○FBS			
Notes:										
	○am. ○pm.						○Pre○Post○FBS			
Notes:										
	○am. ○pm.						○Pre○Post○FBS			
Notes:										
	○am. ○pm.						○Pre○Post○FBS			
Notes:										
	○am. ○pm.						○Pre○Post○FBS			
Notes:										
	○am. ○pm.						○Pre○Post○FBS			
Notes:										
	○am. ○pm.						○Pre○Post○FBS			
Notes:										
	○am. ○pm.						○Pre○Post○FBS			
Notes:										
	○am. ○pm.						○Pre○Post○FBS			
Notes:										
	○am. ○pm.						○Pre○Post○FBS			
Notes:										
	○am. ○pm.						○Pre○Post○FBS			
Notes:										
	○am. ○pm.						○Pre○Post○FBS			

> ....

Month: ....
Year: ....

Date	Time	SYS / DIA (Blood Pressure)	Heart Rate	Respiratory Rate	Oxygen Level	Blood Sugar (Pre/Post Meal or Fasting)	°C / °F (Temperature)	Weight	Notes
	○am. ○pm.					○Pre ○Post ○FBS			
Notes:									
	○am. ○pm.					○Pre ○Post ○FBS			
Notes:									
	○am. ○pm.					○Pre ○Post ○FBS			
Notes:									
	○am. ○pm.					○Pre ○Post ○FBS			
Notes:									
	○am. ○pm.					○Pre ○Post ○FBS			
Notes:									
	○am. ○pm.					○Pre ○Post ○FBS			
Notes:									
	○am. ○pm.					○Pre ○Post ○FBS			
Notes:									
	○am. ○pm.					○Pre ○Post ○FBS			
Notes:									
	○am. ○pm.					○Pre ○Post ○FBS			
Notes:									
	○am. ○pm.					○Pre ○Post ○FBS			
Notes:									
	○am. ○pm.					○Pre ○Post ○FBS			
Notes:									
	○am. ○pm.					○Pre ○Post ○FBS			
Notes:									
	○am. ○pm.					○Pre ○Post ○FBS			
Notes:									
	○am. ○pm.					○Pre ○Post ○FBS			
Notes:									
	○am. ○pm.					○Pre ○Post ○FBS			
Notes:									
	○am. ○pm.					○Pre ○Post ○FBS			

> ....

Month:........................
Year:........................

Date	Time	SYS / DIA	Blood Pressure /	Heart Rate /	Respiratory Rate /	Oxygen Level /	Blood Sugar (Pre/Post Meal or Fasting)	Temperature °C/°F /	Weight	Notes
	○am. ○pm.						○Pre○Post○FBS			
Notes:										
	○am. ○pm.						○Pre○Post○FBS			
Notes:										
	○am. ○pm.						○Pre○Post○FBS			
Notes:										
	○am. ○pm.						○Pre○Post○FBS			
Notes:										
	○am. ○pm.						○Pre○Post○FBS			
Notes:										
	○am. ○pm.						○Pre○Post○FBS			
Notes:										
	○am. ○pm.						○Pre○Post○FBS			
Notes:										
	○am. ○pm.						○Pre○Post○FBS			
Notes:										
	○am. ○pm.						○Pre○Post○FBS			
Notes:										
	○am. ○pm.						○Pre○Post○FBS			
Notes:										
	○am. ○pm.						○Pre○Post○FBS			
Notes:										
	○am. ○pm.						○Pre○Post○FBS			
Notes:										
	○am. ○pm.						○Pre○Post○FBS			
Notes:										
	○am. ○pm.						○Pre○Post○FBS			
Notes:										
	○am. ○pm.						○Pre○Post○FBS			
Notes:										
	○am. ○pm.						○Pre○Post○FBS			

Medication Information

Date	Medication	Notes

Medication Information

Date	Medication	Notes

Medication Information

Date	Medication	Notes

Notes

Notes

Notes

Notes

Notes

> ....

Month: ....
Year: ....

Date	Time	SYS / DIA Blood Pressure	Heart Rate	Respiratory Rate	Oxygen Level	Blood Sugar (Pre/Post Meal or Fasting)	Temperature °C / °F	Weight	Notes
	○am. ○pm.					○Pre ○Post ○FBS			
Notes:									
	○am. ○pm.					○Pre ○Post ○FBS			
Notes:									
	○am. ○pm.					○Pre ○Post ○FBS			
Notes:									
	○am. ○pm.					○Pre ○Post ○FBS			
Notes:									
	○am. ○pm.					○Pre ○Post ○FBS			
Notes:									
	○am. ○pm.					○Pre ○Post ○FBS			
Notes:									
	○am. ○pm.					○Pre ○Post ○FBS			
Notes:									
	○am. ○pm.					○Pre ○Post ○FBS			
Notes:									
	○am. ○pm.					○Pre ○Post ○FBS			
Notes:									
	○am. ○pm.					○Pre ○Post ○FBS			
Notes:									
	○am. ○pm.					○Pre ○Post ○FBS			
Notes:									
	○am. ○pm.					○Pre ○Post ○FBS			
Notes:									
	○am. ○pm.					○Pre ○Post ○FBS			
Notes:									
	○am. ○pm.					○Pre ○Post ○FBS			
Notes:									
	○am. ○pm.					○Pre ○Post ○FBS			
Notes:									
	○am. ○pm.					○Pre ○Post ○FBS			

> ....

Month:........................
Year:........................

Date	Time	SYS / DIA	Blood Pressure /	Heart Rate /	Respiratory Rate /	Oxygen Level /	Blood Sugar (Pre/Post Meal or Fasting)	Temperature °C/°F	Weight /	Notes
	○am. ○pm.						○Pre ○Post ○FBS			
Notes:										
	○am. ○pm.						○Pre ○Post ○FBS			
Notes:										
	○am. ○pm.						○Pre ○Post ○FBS			
Notes:										
	○am. ○pm.						○Pre ○Post ○FBS			
Notes:										
	○am. ○pm.						○Pre ○Post ○FBS			
Notes:										
	○am. ○pm.						○Pre ○Post ○FBS			
Notes:										
	○am. ○pm.						○Pre ○Post ○FBS			
Notes:										
	○am. ○pm.						○Pre ○Post ○FBS			
Notes:										
	○am. ○pm.						○Pre ○Post ○FBS			
Notes:										
	○am. ○pm.						○Pre ○Post ○FBS			
Notes:										
	○am. ○pm.						○Pre ○Post ○FBS			
Notes:										
	○am. ○pm.						○Pre ○Post ○FBS			
Notes:										
	○am. ○pm.						○Pre ○Post ○FBS			
Notes:										
	○am. ○pm.						○Pre ○Post ○FBS			
Notes:										
	○am. ○pm.						○Pre ○Post ○FBS			
Notes:										
	○am. ○pm.						○Pre ○Post ○FBS			

>
....

Month:........................
Year:........................

Date	Time	Blood Pressure SYS / DIA	Heart Rate /	Respiratory Rate /	Oxygen Level /	Blood Sugar (Pre/Post Meal or Fasting) /	Temperature °C / °F	Weight /	Notes
	○am. ○pm.					○Pre ○Post ○FBS			
Notes:									
	○am. ○pm.					○Pre ○Post ○FBS			
Notes:									
	○am. ○pm.					○Pre ○Post ○FBS			
Notes:									
	○am. ○pm.					○Pre ○Post ○FBS			
Notes:									
	○am. ○pm.					○Pre ○Post ○FBS			
Notes:									
	○am. ○pm.					○Pre ○Post ○FBS			
Notes:									
	○am. ○pm.					○Pre ○Post ○FBS			
Notes:									
	○am. ○pm.					○Pre ○Post ○FBS			
Notes:									
	○am. ○pm.					○Pre ○Post ○FBS			
Notes:									
	○am. ○pm.					○Pre ○Post ○FBS			
Notes:									
	○am. ○pm.					○Pre ○Post ○FBS			
Notes:									
	○am. ○pm.					○Pre ○Post ○FBS			
Notes:									
	○am. ○pm.					○Pre ○Post ○FBS			
Notes:									
	○am. ○pm.					○Pre ○Post ○FBS			
Notes:									
	○am. ○pm.					○Pre ○Post ○FBS			
Notes:									
	○am. ○pm.					○Pre ○Post ○FBS			

> ....

Month:..........................
Year:........................

Date	Time	SYS / DIA	Blood Pressure /	Heart Rate /	Respiratory Rate /	Oxygen Level /	Blood Sugar (Pre/Post Meal or Fasting)	Temperature °C/°F	Weight /	Notes
	○am. ○pm.						○Pre○Post○FBS			
Notes:										
	○am. ○pm.						○Pre○Post○FBS			
Notes:										
	○am. ○pm.						○Pre○Post○FBS			
Notes:										
	○am. ○pm.						○Pre○Post○FBS			
Notes:										
	○am. ○pm.						○Pre○Post○FBS			
Notes:										
	○am. ○pm.						○Pre○Post○FBS			
Notes:										
	○am. ○pm.						○Pre○Post○FBS			
Notes:										
	○am. ○pm.						○Pre○Post○FBS			
Notes:										
	○am. ○pm.						○Pre○Post○FBS			
Notes:										
	○am. ○pm.						○Pre○Post○FBS			
Notes:										
	○am. ○pm.						○Pre○Post○FBS			
Notes:										
	○am. ○pm.						○Pre○Post○FBS			
Notes:										
	○am. ○pm.						○Pre○Post○FBS			
Notes:										
	○am. ○pm.						○Pre○Post○FBS			
Notes:										
	○am. ○pm.						○Pre○Post○FBS			
Notes:										
	○am. ○pm.						○Pre○Post○FBS			

\>
....

Month:........................
Year:........................

Date	Time	SYS / DIA	Blood Pressure	Heart Rate	Respiratory Rate	Oxygen Level	Blood Sugar (Pre/Post Meal or Fasting)	Temperature °C/°F	Weight	Notes
	○am. ○pm.						○Pre ○Post ○FBS			
Notes:										
	○am. ○pm.						○Pre ○Post ○FBS			
Notes:										
	○am. ○pm.						○Pre ○Post ○FBS			
Notes:										
	○am. ○pm.						○Pre ○Post ○FBS			
Notes:										
	○am. ○pm.						○Pre ○Post ○FBS			
Notes:										
	○am. ○pm.						○Pre ○Post ○FBS			
Notes:										
	○am. ○pm.						○Pre ○Post ○FBS			
Notes:										
	○am. ○pm.						○Pre ○Post ○FBS			
Notes:										
	○am. ○pm.						○Pre ○Post ○FBS			
Notes:										
	○am. ○pm.						○Pre ○Post ○FBS			
Notes:										
	○am. ○pm.						○Pre ○Post ○FBS			
Notes:										
	○am. ○pm.						○Pre ○Post ○FBS			
Notes:										
	○am. ○pm.						○Pre ○Post ○FBS			
Notes:										
	○am. ○pm.						○Pre ○Post ○FBS			
Notes:										
	○am. ○pm.						○Pre ○Post ○FBS			
Notes:										
	○am. ○pm.						○Pre ○Post ○FBS			

> ....

Month:..........................
Year:........................

Date	Time	SYS / DIA	Blood Pressure	Heart Rate	Respiratory Rate	Oxygen Level	Blood Sugar (Pre/Post Meal or Fasting)	Temperature °C/°F	Weight	Notes
	○am. ○pm.						○Pre ○Post ○FBS			
Notes:										
	○am. ○pm.						○Pre ○Post ○FBS			
Notes:										
	○am. ○pm.						○Pre ○Post ○FBS			
Notes:										
	○am. ○pm.						○Pre ○Post ○FBS			
Notes:										
	○am. ○pm.						○Pre ○Post ○FBS			
Notes:										
	○am. ○pm.						○Pre ○Post ○FBS			
Notes:										
	○am. ○pm.						○Pre ○Post ○FBS			
Notes:										
	○am. ○pm.						○Pre ○Post ○FBS			
Notes:										
	○am. ○pm.						○Pre ○Post ○FBS			
Notes:										
	○am. ○pm.						○Pre ○Post ○FBS			
Notes:										
	○am. ○pm.						○Pre ○Post ○FBS			
Notes:										
	○am. ○pm.						○Pre ○Post ○FBS			
Notes:										
	○am. ○pm.						○Pre ○Post ○FBS			
Notes:										
	○am. ○pm.						○Pre ○Post ○FBS			
Notes:										
	○am. ○pm.						○Pre ○Post ○FBS			
Notes:										
	○am. ○pm.						○Pre ○Post ○FBS			

Medication Information

Date	Medication	Notes

Medication Information

Date	Medication	Notes

Medication Information

Date	Medication	Notes

Notes

Notes

Notes

Notes

Notes

> ....

Month:........................
Year:........................

Date	Time	Blood Pressure SYS / DIA	Heart Rate /	Respiratory Rate /	Oxygen Level /	Blood Sugar (Pre/Post Meal or Fasting)	Temperature °C / °F	Weight /	Notes
	○am. ○pm.					○Pre ○Post ○FBS			
Notes:									
	○am. ○pm.					○Pre ○Post ○FBS			
Notes:									
	○am. ○pm.					○Pre ○Post ○FBS			
Notes:									
	○am. ○pm.					○Pre ○Post ○FBS			
Notes:									
	○am. ○pm.					○Pre ○Post ○FBS			
Notes:									
	○am. ○pm.					○Pre ○Post ○FBS			
Notes:									
	○am. ○pm.					○Pre ○Post ○FBS			
Notes:									
	○am. ○pm.					○Pre ○Post ○FBS			
Notes:									
	○am. ○pm.					○Pre ○Post ○FBS			
Notes:									
	○am. ○pm.					○Pre ○Post ○FBS			
Notes:									
	○am. ○pm.					○Pre ○Post ○FBS			
Notes:									
	○am. ○pm.					○Pre ○Post ○FBS			
Notes:									
	○am. ○pm.					○Pre ○Post ○FBS			
Notes:									
	○am. ○pm.					○Pre ○Post ○FBS			
Notes:									
	○am. ○pm.					○Pre ○Post ○FBS			
Notes:									
	○am. ○pm.					○Pre ○Post ○FBS			

> ....

Month:..........................
Year:..........................

Date	Time	SYS / DIA	Blood Pressure	Heart Rate	Respiratory Rate	Oxygen Level	Blood Sugar (Pre/Post Meal or Fasting)	Temperature °C/°F	Weight	Notes
	○am. ○pm.						○Pre ○Post ○FBS			
Notes:										
	○am. ○pm.						○Pre ○Post ○FBS			
Notes:										
	○am. ○pm.						○Pre ○Post ○FBS			
Notes:										
	○am. ○pm.						○Pre ○Post ○FBS			
Notes:										
	○am. ○pm.						○Pre ○Post ○FBS			
Notes:										
	○am. ○pm.						○Pre ○Post ○FBS			
Notes:										
	○am. ○pm.						○Pre ○Post ○FBS			
Notes:										
	○am. ○pm.						○Pre ○Post ○FBS			
Notes:										
	○am. ○pm.						○Pre ○Post ○FBS			
Notes:										
	○am. ○pm.						○Pre ○Post ○FBS			
Notes:										
	○am. ○pm.						○Pre ○Post ○FBS			
Notes:										
	○am. ○pm.						○Pre ○Post ○FBS			
Notes:										
	○am. ○pm.						○Pre ○Post ○FBS			
Notes:										
	○am. ○pm.						○Pre ○Post ○FBS			
Notes:										
	○am. ○pm.						○Pre ○Post ○FBS			
Notes:										
	○am. ○pm.						○Pre ○Post ○FBS			

Month: ....
Year: ....

Date	Time	SYS / DIA (Blood Pressure)	Heart Rate	Respiratory Rate	Oxygen Level	Blood Sugar (Pre/Post Meal or Fasting)	Temperature °C/°F	Weight	Notes
	○am. ○pm.					○Pre ○Post ○FBS			
Notes:									
	○am. ○pm.					○Pre ○Post ○FBS			
Notes:									
	○am. ○pm.					○Pre ○Post ○FBS			
Notes:									
	○am. ○pm.					○Pre ○Post ○FBS			
Notes:									
	○am. ○pm.					○Pre ○Post ○FBS			
Notes:									
	○am. ○pm.					○Pre ○Post ○FBS			
Notes:									
	○am. ○pm.					○Pre ○Post ○FBS			
Notes:									
	○am. ○pm.					○Pre ○Post ○FBS			
Notes:									
	○am. ○pm.					○Pre ○Post ○FBS			
Notes:									
	○am. ○pm.					○Pre ○Post ○FBS			
Notes:									
	○am. ○pm.					○Pre ○Post ○FBS			
Notes:									
	○am. ○pm.					○Pre ○Post ○FBS			
Notes:									
	○am. ○pm.					○Pre ○Post ○FBS			
Notes:									
	○am. ○pm.					○Pre ○Post ○FBS			
Notes:									
	○am. ○pm.					○Pre ○Post ○FBS			
Notes:									
	○am. ○pm.					○Pre ○Post ○FBS			

Medication Information

Date	Medication	Notes

Notes

Thank you!

WE ARE GLAD THAT YOU PURCHASED OUR BOOK!
PLEASE LET US KNOW HOW WE CAN IMPROVE IT!
YOUR FEEDBACK IS ESSENTIAL TO US.

Contact us at:

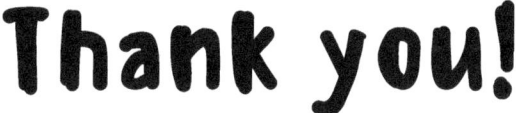 log'Sin@gmail.com

---

JUST TITLE THE EMAIL 'CREATIVE' AND WE WILL GIVE YOU SOME EXTRA SURPRISES!

CPSIA information can be obtained
at www.ICGtesting.com
Printed in the USA
LVHW051307050423
743553LV00006B/167

9 781803 852065